SAXENDA USAGE GU

Comprehensive Insights into Saxenda A Complete Guide to Safe and Effective Weight Management

CONTENT

1. Introduction

2. The science behind saxenda

3. Who should use saxenda

4. Getting started with saxenda

5. Saxenda dosing and administration

6. Lifestyle integration: diet, exercise, and saxenda

7. Side effects and safety precautions

8. Monitoring progress and adjusting the plan

9. Saxenda for specific populations

10. Psychological and emotional aspects of weight loss

11. Alternatives, supplements, and complementary therapies

12. Real stories and expert perspectives

13. Conclusion

INTRODUCTION

Obesity is not merely a condition of excess weight—it is a complex, chronic disease that affects millions of individuals physically, emotionally, and socially. In today's world, where lifestyle, genetics, environmental factors, and mental health all interplay to influence body weight, managing obesity has become an intricate medical and personal challenge. The rise in obesity rates across the globe has brought an urgent need for effective, long-term solutions. The journey toward sustainable weight management extends beyond diet trends and fleeting fitness programs—it demands medically supported, evidence-based interventions tailored to each individual's unique needs.

A. Understanding obesity and chronic weight management

Obesity is now recognized as a chronic disease by major health organizations, including the world health organization and the american medical association. It is characterized by excessive fat accumulation that presents a risk to health, leading to increased susceptibility to conditions such as type 2 diabetes, cardiovascular disease, hypertension, sleep apnea, osteoarthritis, and certain cancers. More importantly, it often carries psychological burdens—low self-esteem, anxiety, and depression.

Chronic weight management is not about temporary fixes; it is about establishing a long-term, sustainable approach to health. This involves a multifaceted strategy that incorporates lifestyle changes, behavioral support, physical activity, nutritional counseling, and, in many cases, medical treatment. Recognizing obesity as a complex and chronic issue allows for a more compassionate, patient-centered approach that prioritizes long-term success over short-term results.

B. The rise of prescription weight loss solutions

Over the past two decades, there has been a growing recognition that traditional weight loss methods—though valuable—often fail to produce lasting results for many individuals struggling with obesity. This has led to increased research and innovation in pharmacological solutions for weight loss. Prescription weight loss medications have emerged as a pivotal component in comprehensive weight management strategies, especially for those who have struggled with conventional methods.

Among these pharmaceutical interventions, glp-1 receptor agonists have shown remarkable promise. These medications mimic the body's natural hormones that regulate appetite, satiety, and glucose metabolism. Saxenda (liraglutide), a prominent glp-1 analog, has been approved specifically for weight management in adults with obesity or overweight individuals with related health conditions. It represents a new frontier in the fight against obesity—a tool that, when used appropriately, can support meaningful, long-term weight reduction.

C. What is saxenda? An overview

Saxenda (liraglutide 3.0 mg) is an fda-approved prescription injectable medication that helps adults and adolescents aged 12 to 17 years with obesity or those who are overweight with weight-related medical problems to lose weight and keep it off. It is not a magic bullet, nor is it a standalone solution. Rather, saxenda is a part of a comprehensive treatment plan that includes a reduced-calorie diet and increased physical activity.

Liraglutide, the active ingredient in saxenda, works by mimicking a hormone called glp-1 that targets areas of the brain involved in appetite regulation and food intake. By helping individuals feel fuller for longer and reducing cravings, saxenda supports behavior changes necessary for long-term weight loss. However, as with any medication, understanding how to use saxenda correctly, manage expectations, recognize side effects, and integrate it into a holistic plan is critical for success.

D. and objectives of this guide

This guide is written with clarity, empathy, and scientific accuracy to empower readers with the knowledge needed to use saxenda safely and effectively. Our goals are multifaceted:

To provide a clear understanding of how saxenda works within the body and its role in managing chronic obesity.

To guide patients through the initiation, dosage adjustment, and maintenance phases of saxenda therapy.

To explore common side effects, strategies to manage them, and signs when medical attention is required.

To emphasize the importance of lifestyle changes, behavioral support, and the role of ongoing medical supervision.

To serve as a resource for healthcare professionals and caregivers in supporting patients on this journey.

This guide seeks to educate, encourage, and equip readers with the tools they need to achieve better health outcomes through informed choices.

E. Who this book is for: patients, caregivers, and healthcare providers

This book is written for a broad and diverse audience:

Patients who are beginning or considering saxenda therapy will find detailed, compassionate guidance to help them understand the process and what to expect.

Caregivers who support loved ones dealing with obesity will benefit from insights into the treatment process and learn how to provide meaningful, empathetic assistance.

Healthcare providers—whether physicians, nurse practitioners, pharmacists, or dietitians—will find this guide useful as a supplementary tool in educating and counseling their patients.

Whether you are on your personal journey to better health, assisting someone you care for, or helping patients professionally, this guide aims to bridge the gap between medical expertise and everyday experience. Our approach is rooted in evidence-based information and practical advice, with the ultimate goal of transforming knowledge into positive, measurable outcomes.

Welcome to the saxenda usage guide—a comprehensive, reliable resource to help you navigate the path toward healthier weight and a healthier life.

THE SCIENCE BEHIND SAXENDA

Understanding the science of how saxenda works is essential for patients, caregivers, and healthcare providers seeking to make informed decisions about weight loss therapy. Saxenda (liraglutide) represents a powerful tool in the fight against obesity, but its success lies in its biological mechanisms, how it compares with other medications, and the strong clinical evidence behind its use. This chapter explores the foundation of saxenda's effectiveness by examining the critical scientific principles that drive its action.

A. How saxenda works: the role of glp-1 receptor agonists

Saxenda is a glp-1 receptor agonist, a class of medications originally developed to manage type 2 diabetes. Glp-1, or glucagon-like peptide-1, is a naturally occurring hormone that plays a key role in appetite regulation and glucose metabolism.

After eating, glp-1 is released in the gut, where it binds to receptors in the pancreas, brain, and gastrointestinal tract. This hormone promotes insulin secretion in response to elevated blood glucose and reduces the secretion of glucagon (a hormone that raises blood sugar). More importantly for weight loss, glp-1 signals to the brain—particularly to the hypothalamus—that the body is full, leading to reduced appetite and increased satiety.

Saxenda mimics the effects of natural glp-1 but has a longer half-life, meaning it stays active in the body longer and provides sustained effects on appetite suppression and blood sugar control. Administered via daily subcutaneous injection, saxenda works continuously to help patients reduce food intake without significantly altering their metabolic rate or causing excessive hunger or weakness.

B. Saxenda vs. Other weight loss medications

The landscape of weight loss medications has expanded significantly, and comparing saxenda with alternatives like ozempic, wegovy, contrave, and phentermine helps clarify its unique benefits and limitations.

Ozempic (semaglutide) and wegovy (also semaglutide) are also glp-1 receptor agonists. While ozempic is approved primarily for type 2 diabetes and is dosed weekly, wegovy is approved for chronic weight management. Wegovy delivers higher doses of semaglutide than ozempic, resulting in greater weight loss outcomes. Compared to saxenda, semaglutide has a longer duration of action and may offer greater weight reduction, but saxenda remains a viable option for those needing daily glp-1 administration or those sensitive to semaglutide's side effect profile.

Contrave combines bupropion (an antidepressant) and naltrexone (used in addiction treatment). It acts on the central nervous system to reduce food cravings and increase energy expenditure. However, it has a different side effect profile and interacts with more medications, making saxenda a preferable choice for patients requiring glucose regulation support.

Phentermine, one of the oldest weight loss drugs, is a stimulant that suppresses appetite via norepinephrine release in the brain. While effective for short-term use, it is not approved for long-term management and carries risks such as increased heart rate, dependence, and insomnia. Saxenda, by contrast, is suitable for long-term, sustainable weight loss with a different safety profile.

In summary, saxenda offers a non-stimulant, hormone-based approach to weight management, focusing on appetite control through physiological pathways rather than central nervous system stimulation or mood alteration.

C. Understanding appetite regulation and satiety

To appreciate saxenda's effectiveness, it is essential to understand the neuroendocrine regulation of appetite. Hunger and fullness are governed by a complex interplay of hormones and brain regions—particularly the hypothalamus and brainstem.

Key hormones involved include:

Ghrelin, known as the "hunger hormone," is produced in the stomach and signals the brain to initiate eating.

Leptin, produced by fat cells, suppresses hunger and promotes energy balance.

Glp-1, the hormone mimicked by saxenda, enhances the sensation of fullness and slows gastric emptying, which contributes to longer-lasting satiety after meals.

Saxenda effectively modulates the brain's reward and appetite centers, helping patients feel full sooner and for longer periods. By reducing the frequency and volume of food intake without compromising nutritional adequacy, saxenda supports a healthy caloric deficit, a cornerstone of weight loss.

    D.   The impact of saxenda on metabolism and insulin regulation

Though saxenda is not classified as a diabetes medication in its weight-loss formulation, its active ingredient—liraglutide—has significant benefits for glucose metabolism and insulin sensitivity.

Patients with insulin resistance, prediabetes, or metabolic syndrome often find it difficult to lose weight because insulin's fat-storing effects interfere with the breakdown of body fat. Saxenda improves this by:

Enhancing insulin secretion in a glucose-dependent manner (only when blood sugar is elevated),

Reducing glucagon secretion, thus lowering fasting and post-meal blood glucose,

Delaying gastric emptying, which slows the rate at which glucose enters the bloodstream.

These actions reduce insulin spikes, minimize fat storage, and promote improved metabolic efficiency. In individuals with elevated fasting glucose or early type 2 diabetes, saxenda often contributes to better glycemic control alongside weight loss—an outcome that benefits cardiovascular and endocrine health.

E. Fda approval and clinical trials: evidence-based results

Saxenda received fda approval in december 2014 for chronic weight management in adults with a body mass index (bmi) of:

≥30 kg/m² (obesity), or

≥27 kg/m² (overweight) with at least one weight-related condition (e.g., hypertension, dyslipidemia, or type 2 diabetes).

Approval was based on a series of robust phase 3 clinical trials, including the scale (satiety and clinical adiposity–liraglutide evidence) studies, which involved more than 4,800 participants.

Key findings from these trials include:

Average weight loss of 8-10% of initial body weight after one year, significantly more than with placebo.

Improvement in cardiometabolic markers, including blood pressure, cholesterol levels, and fasting blood glucose.

Reduced risk of progression to type 2 diabetes in individuals with prediabetes.

Moreover, participants reported greater satisfaction with eating behavior, improved emotional well-being, and increased motivation to adopt healthy lifestyle habits when using saxenda compared to placebo groups.

Safety data from these trials showed that most side effects were gastrointestinal in nature (nausea, vomiting, diarrhea), typically resolving over time. The risk of serious adverse events was low, though patients must be screened for contraindications such as a history of medullary thyroid carcinoma or pancreatitis.

WHO SHOULD USE SAXENDA

Saxenda (liraglutide 3.0 mg) is a prescription medication approved as an adjunct to a reduced-calorie diet and increased physical activity for chronic weight management. Understanding who should use saxenda—and who should not—is essential for ensuring its safe, effective, and medically appropriate use. This section explores the indications for use, eligibility criteria, potential candidates with comorbidities like type 2 diabetes, contraindications, and the critical role of professional medical evaluation before starting therapy.

A. Indications for use: adults and adolescents (12–17 years)

Saxenda is primarily indicated for:

Adults with a body mass index (bmi) of 30 kg/m² or greater (classified as obese), or

Adults with a bmi of 27 kg/m² or greater (overweight) and at least one weight-related comorbid condition, such as hypertension, dyslipidemia, or type 2 diabetes mellitus.

Additionally, saxenda is approved for use in adolescents aged 12–17 years with:

A body weight above 60 kg (132 pounds), and

An initial bmi corresponding to 30 kg/m² or greater for adults, adjusted for age and sex using standardized growth charts.

Saxenda is not intended for general weight loss or cosmetic purposes; it is a medically supervised intervention for those who meet clinical criteria and require pharmacological support for weight management.

B. Bmi thresholds and eligibility criteria

Eligibility for saxenda is closely linked to bmi classifications:

Obese adults (bmi ≥ 30 kg/m²) qualify regardless of comorbidities.

Overweight adults (bmi ≥ 27 kg/m²) must present at least one obesity-related condition, such as:

Type 2 diabetes

Cardiovascular disease

Obstructive sleep apnea

Polycystic ovary syndrome (pcos)

Non-alcoholic fatty liver disease (nafld)

Adolescents must meet age-appropriate bmi percentiles as outlined by the cdc or who growth charts and should be under pediatric care for comprehensive evaluation.

Saxenda should be considered only when lifestyle modification alone has proven insufficient, and when the potential benefits outweigh the risks.

C. Saxenda for patients with type 2 diabetes

Saxenda is often prescribed to adults with type 2 diabetes who also struggle with weight management. Weight loss in these patients can improve glycemic control, reduce the need for additional antidiabetic medications, and lower cardiovascular risk.

Although liraglutide is also sold under the brand name victoza at a lower dose for glycemic management, saxenda is specifically formulated and dosed for weight loss. Patients with type 2 diabetes may benefit from saxenda in several ways:

Improved insulin sensitivity

Decreased hba1c levels

Lower fasting glucose

Reduction in visceral fat

However, saxenda is not a substitute for diabetes medication and should be used in conjunction with appropriate antidiabetic therapy under medical supervision.

D. Who should not use saxenda: contraindications and warnings

Not all individuals are appropriate candidates for saxenda. Contraindications include:

Personal or family history of medullary thyroid carcinoma (mtc)

Patients with multiple endocrine neoplasia syndrome type 2 (men 2)

Pregnancy and breastfeeding

Known hypersensitivity to liraglutide or any components of the formulation

Caution is also advised in individuals with:

A history of pancreatitis

Gallbladder disease

Severe gastrointestinal disorders, especially gastroparesis

Depression or suicidal thoughts (patients should be monitored for mood changes)

Severe renal or hepatic impairment

Using saxenda outside the recommended guidelines can lead to serious adverse effects. Its use should be strictly limited to those for whom the potential benefits outweigh the risks, and in accordance with clinical standards.

E. Consultation and evaluation: the importance of medical supervision

Before initiating saxenda therapy, a comprehensive medical evaluation is essential. This includes:

Baseline weight and bmi measurements

Screening for comorbid conditions such as diabetes, cardiovascular disease, and hormonal disorders

Assessment of contraindications

Discussion of lifestyle interventions and long-term weight management strategies

Monitoring plans for side effects, progress, and goals

Because saxenda is a prescription-only medication, it must be initiated and managed by a qualified healthcare provider. Ongoing follow-up ensures that the patient responds appropriately and tolerates the treatment well. This also allows for timely adjustments or discontinuation if needed.

Healthcare providers may also collaborate with dietitians, fitness professionals, and behavioral health specialists to support a comprehensive and sustainable weight management plan.

GETTING STARTED WITH SAXENDA

Embarking on a weight loss journey with saxenda is not simply about taking an injection—it's a holistic commitment to improving your health, reshaping your lifestyle, and understanding your body's needs. Whether you've struggled with weight management for years or are just beginning to explore medical options, this section will guide you through the essential steps before and during your initiation with saxenda.

A. Preparing for your weight loss journey

Before you take your first dose of saxenda, it's important to mentally and physically prepare yourself for what lies ahead. Saxenda is a tool—an effective one—but lasting weight loss involves behavioral change, dietary improvement, and increased physical activity.

Start by reflecting on your motivation. Are you seeking to prevent or manage health conditions like type 2 diabetes, high blood pressure, or sleep apnea? Are you aiming for better mobility, energy, or self-esteem? Clarifying your reasons provides a strong foundation when challenges arise.

Prepare your environment by removing tempting, high-calorie foods and replacing them with nutritious alternatives. Schedule time for daily walks or physical activity you enjoy. Talk to your support network—friends, family, or a weight-loss group—and let them know you're beginning a medically guided weight loss journey. Emotional and practical support will be invaluable along the way.

B. Initial medical assessment and health history

Before starting saxenda, a comprehensive medical assessment by a licensed healthcare provider is essential.

Saxenda (liraglutide) is approved for adults with a body mass index (bmi) of:

30 or higher (obesity), or

27 or higher (overweight) with at least one weight-related health condition such as hypertension, type 2 diabetes, or dyslipidemia.

Your healthcare provider will evaluate your health history to ensure saxenda is a safe and suitable option. This includes reviewing:

Past and current medical conditions, especially thyroid issues, pancreatitis, gallbladder disease, or depression.

Family history, especially of medullary thyroid carcinoma (mtc) or multiple endocrine neoplasia syndrome type 2 (men 2).

Current medications, as interactions may exist, particularly with insulin or other glp-1 receptor agonists.

Weight loss attempts, including diets, exercise, and other medications or surgeries.

Mental health history, since mood changes, depression, and suicidal thoughts are risks that must be monitored closely.

Lab work may be ordered to assess your baseline blood sugar levels, thyroid function, liver function, and other markers that will help monitor your progress and safety during treatment.

C. How to obtain a prescription: steps to access

To start saxenda, follow these key steps:

Schedule a visit with a licensed healthcare provider: this could be your primary care physician, an endocrinologist, or an obesity medicine specialist.

Request a weight loss evaluation: be honest about your struggles and interest in medical treatment. Bring any documentation of previous attempts at weight loss.

Discuss your eligibility: based on your bmi, health status, and lifestyle, your provider will determine if saxenda is appropriate.

Prescription and education: if approved, your provider will write a prescription and educate you on dosing, administration (via subcutaneous injection), and side effects.

Pharmacy fulfillment: most pharmacies carry saxenda, but availability may vary. Your provider or a specialty pharmacy may help coordinate access, especially if prior authorization is needed.

If you're uncomfortable with self-injection, ask your provider for a demonstration or referral to a diabetes educator or nurse practitioner for training.

    D.   Insurance coverage, costs, and patient assistance programs

Saxenda can be expensive—costs may exceed $1,000 per month without insurance. Fortunately, there are several avenues to make it more affordable:

Check your insurance plan: many private insurers and some medicaid plans may cover saxenda with prior authorization. Your provider will likely need to submit documentation supporting medical necessity.

Saxenda savings card: novo nordisk offers a savings card for eligible patients, significantly lowering out-of-pocket costs for those with commercial insurance.

Patient assistance program (pap): for those without insurance or with financial hardship, novo nordisk's pap may provide saxenda at no cost. Visit the company's official website or ask your provider's office for help applying.

Pharmacy discounts: check discount programs like goodrx, although savings may be limited for brand-name drugs.

Ensure you follow up with your provider's office to handle insurance appeals or documentation, as persistence is often necessary to get coverage approved.

E. Setting realistic goals and expectations

Starting saxenda with realistic expectations is key to long-term success. Saxenda is not a magic bullet; it's a scientifically backed tool designed to help you control hunger and make lifestyle changes easier.

Clinical trials show that with saxenda, patients often lose 5% to 10% of their starting body weight within six months to a year. These outcomes assume consistent medication use, dietary improvements, and increased physical activity. Remember, even modest weight loss—5% of your body weight—can significantly improve blood pressure, blood sugar, cholesterol, and joint pain.

Discuss your goals with your healthcare provider and set milestones:

Short-term goals: examples include taking your injections consistently for the first month, reducing fast food intake, or walking 20 minutes daily.

Long-term goals: these may include reaching a target weight range, lowering a1c levels, or reducing the need for medications.

Track your progress not just on the scale, but through how your clothes fit, your energy levels, sleep quality, and mood. Celebrate every achievement, no matter how small.

SAXENDA DOSING AND ADMINISTRATION

Saxenda (liraglutide 3 mg) is a prescription injectable medication used for chronic weight management in adults with obesity or overweight and at least one weight-related condition. Proper dosing and administration are crucial to ensure its effectiveness and reduce the risk of side effects. This section offers a comprehensive overview of how to use saxenda safely and effectively, including how to inject it, titrate the dose, choose injection sites, reduce discomfort, and manage the storage and disposal of the pen device.

A. Step-by-step guide to injection

Administering saxenda is a straightforward process when following a systematic approach. It is a once-daily subcutaneous injection, and it's essential to follow these steps each time:

Wash your hands

Begin by thoroughly washing your hands with soap and water to reduce the risk of infection.

Check the pen

Remove the saxenda pen cap and inspect the solution. It should be clear and colorless. Do not use it if the solution is cloudy, colored, or contains particles.

Attach a new needle

Peel off the protective seal from a new disposable needle and screw it firmly onto the pen. Remove the outer and inner needle caps.

Check the flow (priming)

If you're using a new pen or haven't used it in a while, perform a flow check to ensure the medication is dispensing correctly. Turn the dose selector to the flow check symbol (usually indicated) and press the injection button until a drop appears at the needle tip.

Select the dose

Turn the dose selector to the correct dose as prescribed by your healthcare provider (see titration schedule below). Make sure the dose window shows the correct number before injecting.

Choose an injection site

Use a recommended subcutaneous site (abdomen, thigh, or upper arm).

Inject the medication

Pinch the skin gently to lift the fatty tissue, insert the needle at a 90-degree angle, and press the injection button all the way down. Hold the pen in place for at least 6 seconds to ensure full delivery of the dose.

Withdraw and dispose of the needle

Remove the needle from the skin, place the outer needle cap back on, unscrew it, and safely dispose of it in a sharps container.

Store the pen properly

Replace the pen cap and return the pen to proper storage conditions immediately.

B. Saxenda dose titration schedule

To minimize gastrointestinal side effects such as nausea and vomiting, saxenda dosing must be increased gradually. This titration approach allows the body to adjust to the medication over time:

Week 1: 0.6 mg once daily

Week 2: 1.2 mg once daily

Week 3: 1.8 mg once daily

Week 4: 2.4 mg once daily

Week 5 and onward: 3.0 mg once daily (maintenance dose)

Your healthcare provider may adjust the titration schedule based on how well you tolerate each dose. If side effects become problematic, a slower escalation or temporary dose reduction may be advised. Do not exceed the maximum dose of 3.0 mg per day.

C. Recommended injection sites and techniques

Saxenda is administered via subcutaneous (under the skin) injection. The following sites are considered safe and effective:

Abdomen (stomach area): at least 2 inches away from the navel, avoiding scars or irritated skin.

Front of the thighs: approximately midway between the hip and the knee.

Upper arm: the fleshy area on the back of the arm (requires assistance or careful technique if self-administering).

Best practices:

Rotate injection sites within the same region to prevent lipodystrophy (changes in fat tissue).

Do not inject into veins or muscles.

Avoid areas that are tender, bruised, red, or hard.

Use a firm, steady motion to insert the needle, and do not rush the injection.

D. Tips to reduce injection discomfort

While most people tolerate saxenda injections well, mild discomfort or skin irritation can occur. These tips may help minimize pain and improve the experience:

Use a new needle for each injection to maintain sharpness and hygiene.

Let the medication reach room temperature before injecting, if stored in the refrigerator.

Relax the muscle at the injection site to avoid unnecessary tension.

Pinch the skin gently and insert the needle quickly but steadily.

Inject slowly and steadily to reduce tissue pressure.

Apply a cool compress or gentle massage after injection if mild soreness develops.

Avoid injecting in the same exact spot repeatedly.

If severe pain, bleeding, or bruising occurs frequently, consult your healthcare provider to rule out incorrect technique or needle size issues.

E. Safe storage, handling, and disposal of pens

Proper storage and handling of saxenda pens are essential for maintaining medication integrity and user safety.

Storage:

Before first use: store the pen in a refrigerator at 36°f to 46°f (2°c to 8°c). Do not freeze. Discard the pen if it has been frozen.

After first use: the pen may be stored at room temperature (59°f to 86°f or 15°c to 30°c) or in the refrigerator. Keep the pen away from heat and sunlight.

Use the pen within 30 days of first use. Discard any unused medication after this period, even if some remains.

Handling:

Always attach a new, sterile needle before each injection.

Never share your pen with others, even if the needle is changed.

Do not use if the pen has been dropped or appears damaged.

Disposal:

Dispose of used needles in a puncture-resistant sharps container. Never throw loose needles in the trash.

When the pen is empty, remove the needle and dispose of the pen according to local regulations or pharmacy take-back programs.

Keep pens and sharps containers out of reach of children and pets.

LIFESTYLE INTEGRATION: DIET, EXERCISE, AND SAXENDA

Saxenda (liraglutide) is not a magic solution—it is a clinically proven aid that works best when integrated into a holistic, sustainable lifestyle. The key pillars of long-term success include mindful nutrition, consistent physical activity, emotional regulation, and continuous self-awareness. In this section, we will explore how to construct a sustainable lifestyle around saxenda, one that supports not just weight loss, but also metabolic health, emotional well-being, and improved quality of life.

A. Nutrition guidelines to complement saxenda use

Saxenda helps to regulate appetite and reduce food intake by interacting with appetite centers in the brain and slowing gastric emptying. To fully capitalize on these effects, dietary choices should align with health-focused principles that support weight management and overall well-being:

1. Prioritize whole, nutrient-dense foods

Consume foods that nourish the body with essential vitamins, minerals, and fiber while minimizing empty calories. Emphasize:

Lean proteins (chicken, turkey, fish, tofu, legumes)

High-fiber vegetables and fruits (spinach, broccoli, berries, apples)

Whole grains (quinoa, oats, brown rice)

Healthy fats (avocados, olive oil, nuts, seeds)

2. Control portion sizes

Saxenda can decrease appetite, but it's still crucial to practice portion control to stay within calorie goals. Use smaller plates, chew thoroughly, and pause during meals to assess satiety.

3. Limit processed foods and added sugars

Avoid sugary beverages, fried foods, packaged snacks, and high-fat fast foods. These contribute excess calories and may counteract the appetite-reducing effects of saxenda.

4. Stay hydrated

Water supports metabolism, digestion, and satiety. Aim for at least 8 cups (2 liters) of water daily. Herbal teas or infused water can provide variety.

5. Time your meals wisely

Some users find success with regular meal timing or intermittent fasting. Consider spacing meals evenly throughout the day to maintain blood sugar stability and manage hunger cues effectively.

B. Sample meal plans and calorie goals

Calorie needs vary based on age, sex, weight, activity level, and health conditions. However, general guidance for weight loss is a reduction of 500–750 calories/day from maintenance levels, often leading to a goal range of 1,200–1,800 calories/day for most adults.

Here is a sample 1,500-calorie day for a person on saxenda:

Breakfast (350 calories):

2 scrambled eggs with spinach and tomatoes

1 slice whole-grain toast

1 small apple

Black coffee or green tea

Snack (100 calories):

10 almonds

Lunch (400 calories):

Grilled chicken breast (4 oz)

Mixed greens salad with olive oil and vinegar

½ cup quinoa

Cucumber and cherry tomato slices

Snack (150 calories):

Greek yogurt (plain, non-fat) with cinnamon

Dinner (500 calories):

Baked salmon (5 oz)

Steamed broccoli and carrots

½ cup sweet potato

Lemon water

Tips:

Track intake using a food journal or app like myfitnesspal.

Adjust portions based on individual hunger levels and saxenda's appetite-suppressing effects.

Consider consulting a registered dietitian for personalized meal planning.

C. Exercise recommendations: from walking to strength training

Exercise enhances the effectiveness of saxenda by accelerating fat loss, preserving lean muscle mass, improving insulin sensitivity, and boosting mood.

1. Start where you are: low-intensity movement

For beginners or those with limited mobility, start with low-impact activities like:

Walking – 20–30 minutes daily, gradually increasing pace and duration

Swimming or water aerobics – gentle on joints and effective for calorie burning

Chair exercises or light yoga – ideal for those recovering from injuries

2. Build up: moderate cardiovascular exercise

Aim for 150–300 minutes/week of moderate-intensity cardio such as:

Brisk walking

Cycling

Dance fitness

Hiking

3. Add strength training (2–3 times per week):

Resistance training builds lean muscle, which boosts basal metabolic rate and helps prevent weight regain.

Bodyweight exercises: squats, push-ups, lunges

Resistance bands or dumbbells: bicep curls, shoulder presses, rows

Core work: planks, crunches, leg lifts

    4. Be consistent, not perfect

Even small bursts of movement throughout the day can add up. Find activities you enjoy and set realistic, achievable fitness goals.

    D.   The importance of behavior change and tracking progress

Sustainable weight management requires more than temporary effort—it demands long-term behavior change, supported by consistent self-monitoring and goal setting.

1. Set smart goals:

Specific: walk 30 minutes daily

Measurable: track meals 5 days/week

Achievable: begin with 10-minute walks

Relevant: improve energy and sleep

Time-bound: lose 5 pounds in 1 month

2. Use tracking tools:

Mobile apps to monitor food, exercise, and weight

Journals for emotional eating and thought patterns

Weekly weigh-ins and waist measurements

3. Create an accountability system:

Support from friends, family, or a health coach

Join online communities or local wellness groups

Celebrate milestones without using food as a reward

E. Emotional eating and mindful eating techniques

Weight challenges often have an emotional dimension. Saxenda helps reduce hunger, but it doesn't remove the psychological triggers that drive emotional eating. Understanding and reprogramming these habits is essential.

1. Recognize triggers:

Stress, boredom, loneliness, fatigue

Environmental cues like watching tv or passing a bakery

Social settings with food pressure

2. Mindful eating practices:

Pause before eating: ask, "am i physically hungry?"

Slow down: chew thoroughly and set utensils down between bites

Eat without distraction: avoid eating in front of screens

Savor food: notice texture, flavor, aroma, and satisfaction level

3. Develop healthy coping mechanisms:

Journaling thoughts and emotions

Engaging in hobbies, creative arts, or nature walks

Practicing deep breathing, meditation, or mindfulness apps

    4. Seek support if needed:

If emotional eating persists, consider cognitive-behavioral therapy (cbt), which is effective in identifying and reshaping unhealthy eating patterns.

SIDE EFFECTS AND SAFETY PRECAUTIONS

When embarking on a weight management journey with saxenda (liraglutide), understanding the full scope of potential side effects and the necessary safety precautions is essential. While saxenda has proven effective for many individuals in reducing weight and improving associated metabolic conditions, it is not without its physiological risks and effects. Being well-informed not only ensures safer usage but also empowers users to respond appropriately to emerging symptoms. This chapter offers a comprehensive exploration of both common and rare side effects, how to manage them, and critical safety considerations every patient should observe.

A. Common side effects: nausea, vomiting, constipation

The majority of individuals using saxenda will encounter mild to moderate side effects, particularly during the initial phase of treatment or when the dosage is increased. The most frequently reported side effects include:

1. Nausea:

Nausea is the most common initial reaction to saxenda, often occurring as the body adapts to the medication. This symptom typically diminishes over time but may return with dosage escalations. Eating smaller, low-fat meals and avoiding rich or spicy foods can help mitigate nausea.

2. Vomiting:

Though less common than nausea, vomiting may occur, especially when the gastrointestinal tract is significantly stimulated. This can lead to dehydration if persistent. Patients should ensure adequate fluid intake and consult their provider if vomiting becomes frequent or severe.

3. Constipation:

Changes in bowel habits are also a recognized effect of saxenda, with constipation being the most common. A fiber-rich diet, increased hydration, and regular physical activity often alleviate this issue. In some cases, a mild over-the-counter laxative may be recommended by a healthcare provider.

These side effects are usually not dangerous but can be uncomfortable. Patients should be encouraged to remain patient during the adjustment phase and use supportive strategies to manage symptoms.

B. Rare but serious side effects: thyroid tumors, pancreatitis, gallbladder issues

Though rare, saxenda has been associated with certain serious adverse effects. These risks should be discussed thoroughly with a healthcare provider prior to starting the medication.

    1. Thyroid c-cell tumors:

Animal studies have indicated an increased risk of thyroid c-cell tumors, including medullary thyroid carcinoma (mtc), in rodents exposed to liraglutide. Although a direct causal relationship in humans has not been established, individuals with a personal or family history of mtc or multiple endocrine neoplasia syndrome type 2 (men 2) should not use saxenda. Symptoms such as a neck lump, hoarseness, difficulty swallowing, or persistent neck pain warrant immediate medical evaluation.

2. Pancreatitis:

Liraglutide has been linked in rare cases to acute pancreatitis, a serious and potentially life-threatening condition. Patients should be educated about signs of pancreatitis, including persistent severe abdominal pain that may radiate to the back, accompanied by vomiting. Discontinuation of saxenda is necessary if pancreatitis is suspected or confirmed.

3. Gallbladder issues:

Rapid weight loss and certain glp-1 receptor agonists, including saxenda, may increase the risk of gallbladder problems such as gallstones or cholecystitis (inflammation of the gallbladder). Symptoms include right upper abdominal pain, nausea, vomiting, and fever. Prompt medical evaluation is critical if these symptoms develop.

C. How to manage side effects effectively

Proactive management is key to maintaining treatment adherence and minimizing discomfort. Below are some strategies for managing side effects:

Titrate gradually: always follow the prescribed titration schedule to allow the body to adjust slowly to the medication.

Dietary adjustments: small, frequent meals; reduced fat intake; and avoiding alcohol can reduce gastrointestinal side effects.

Hydration: drinking adequate fluids helps with both nausea and constipation.

Lifestyle habits: regular physical activity not only supports weight loss but also promotes bowel regularity and mental well-being.

Monitoring: maintain a daily journal of symptoms to track trends and share with your healthcare provider for better clinical management.

Medication aids: over-the-counter remedies, like antiemetics or mild laxatives, may be used with professional guidance.

D. When to contact a healthcare provider

While mild side effects may resolve on their own, certain signs and symptoms require immediate medical attention. Contact a healthcare provider if any of the following occur:

Severe or persistent nausea and vomiting

Intense abdominal pain (especially radiating to the back)

Signs of dehydration (dry mouth, dizziness, decreased urination)

Rapid heartbeat or palpitations

Difficulty breathing or swallowing

Lump or swelling in the neck

Jaundice (yellowing of the skin or eyes)

Signs of allergic reaction (rash, itching, swelling of face/tongue/throat)

Even in the absence of serious symptoms, patients should maintain routine follow-ups to assess tolerance and effectiveness, and adjust dosage as necessary.

E. Drug interactions and medication conflicts

Saxenda may interact with other medications, potentially altering its effects or increasing the risk of adverse reactions. It is vital to inform your healthcare provider of all medications, supplements, and herbal products being used. Notable interactions include:

Insulin and insulin secretagogues (e.g., sulfonylureas): may increase the risk of hypoglycemia. Dosages may need adjustment.

Other glp-1 receptor agonists: concomitant use is not recommended due to overlapping mechanisms and potential toxicity.

Delayed gastric emptying drugs: saxenda slows gastric emptying, which may interfere with the absorption of oral medications, including some antibiotics and pain relievers.

Oral contraceptives: while not contraindicated, delayed gastric emptying could theoretically affect absorption.

Additional birth control methods may be considered during early treatment phases.

Always review medication lists during appointments and be cautious when starting any new drug.

MONITORING PROGRESS AND ADJUSTING THE PLAN

Effective weight loss with saxenda is not a set-it-and-forget-it approach. It is a dynamic journey that requires thoughtful monitoring, ongoing assessment, and strategic adjustment. Success with saxenda is best achieved through a combination of medication, lifestyle changes, and consistent evaluation of progress. This chapter provides a comprehensive framework to help users stay on track, troubleshoot challenges, and ultimately transition into long-term weight maintenance.

A. Tools for tracking weight, appetite, and lifestyle changes

Tracking progress is a cornerstone of effective saxenda use. By collecting accurate and meaningful data, users can identify trends, recognize achievements, and intervene early if progress stalls.

1. Weight tracking tools:

Digital scales with apps: devices such as smart scales can automatically log daily weight and calculate bmi and body fat percentage. These can sync with mobile apps like myfitnesspal, fitbit, or apple health.

Manual logs: a simple paper journal or spreadsheet can serve as a daily tracker for those preferring non-digital options.

Weekly weigh-ins: to avoid fixation on daily fluctuations, some users benefit from weekly rather than daily weigh-ins.

2. Appetite and satiety monitoring:

Hunger scales: using a 1–10 hunger/fullness scale before and after meals can help monitor saxenda's effects on appetite regulation.

Food journaling: logging meals, portion sizes, hunger cues, and emotional eating patterns offers insight into behavioral triggers.

3. Physical activity and lifestyle metrics:

Fitness trackers: devices like garmin, apple watch, or fitbit record steps, workouts, heart rate, and calorie expenditure.

Mood and sleep logs: since saxenda may influence mood and energy, tracking emotional well-being and sleep quality helps assess overall lifestyle improvement.

Behavioral apps: apps such as noom or lose it! Can help monitor habits, set daily goals, and reinforce behavioral change.

The integration of multiple tracking tools paints a clearer picture of your journey, helping healthcare providers make informed decisions and offering the user tangible proof of progress.

B. Importance of regular medical follow-ups

Ongoing communication with your healthcare provider is essential to ensure that saxenda remains effective, safe, and suitable for your personal health profile.

1. Monitoring health parameters:

Vital signs and lab work: regular checks on blood pressure, blood glucose, cholesterol levels, and thyroid function are key to identifying improvements or emerging concerns.

Adverse reactions: monitoring for side effects such as nausea, vomiting, gallbladder issues, or pancreatitis allows for timely intervention.

2. Medication review:

Dose titration: saxenda dosage is gradually increased during initiation. Medical supervision ensures the correct titration schedule based on tolerability and effect.

Drug interactions: as other medications may be added or removed, ongoing review is necessary to avoid negative interactions.

3. Emotional and psychological support:

Mental health monitoring: emotional wellbeing is a vital part of the journey. Healthcare providers can identify and manage issues such as body image distress or eating disorders.

Referral to support services: nutritionists, therapists, or weight management specialists may be recommended for additional guidance.

These regular check-ins provide accountability, allow for recalibration of strategies, and strengthen the patient-provider alliance.

C. Dealing with plateaus and motivation slumps

Weight loss plateaus and dips in motivation are natural and expected phases in any weight management journey. How you respond to them can determine your long-term success.

1. Understanding plateaus:

Metabolic adaptation: as weight decreases, so does basal metabolic rate. This requires adjustments in calorie intake or activity.

Behavioral drift: over time, individuals may become less vigilant with their eating habits or exercise routines.

Hormonal adjustments: hormones affecting hunger and metabolism may rebalance, slowing weight loss.

2. Strategies to overcome plateaus:

Reassess caloric needs: a registered dietitian can help recalculate dietary goals to match your new weight.

Revamp exercise routines: introducing resistance training or increasing intensity may help break plateaus.

Refocus on sleep and stress: sleep deprivation and chronic stress can hinder weight loss.

3. Addressing motivation slumps:

Celebrate non-scale victories: focus on improved clothing fit, stamina, mental clarity, or health markers.

Set mini-goals: break the journey into smaller, achievable milestones to sustain motivation.

Join a support group: peer encouragement, whether in person or online, can provide fresh energy.

D. Adjusting dosage or stopping use safely

Saxenda is not intended for indefinite use without evaluation. Depending on individual response, health outcomes, and tolerability, changes in dosage or discontinuation may be warranted.

1. Adjusting dosage:

Side effect management: if gastrointestinal symptoms become unmanageable, the dose may be reduced or the titration slowed.

Suboptimal results: if expected weight loss is not achieved at the full dose, reassessing lifestyle factors is necessary before increasing or stopping medication.

2. Discontinuing saxenda:

Tapering off: it is advisable to taper rather than abruptly stop to avoid appetite rebound or gastrointestinal discomfort.

Professional supervision: discontinuation should always be discussed with a healthcare provider to ensure a safe transition and to develop a post-medication strategy.

3. Indicators for stopping:

Achieved weight goal: if goal weight is reached and stable, it may be time to transition to maintenance.

Persistent side effects: if adverse effects outweigh benefits, a discontinuation plan should be implemented.

Ineffectiveness: if no significant weight loss occurs after 16 weeks at the full dose, discontinuation is usually recommended.

E. Transitioning to maintenance after goal weight is reached

Reaching your goal weight is a major milestone, but sustaining that weight requires a thoughtful, proactive maintenance plan.

1. Establishing new habits as norms:

Permanent lifestyle changes: continue the healthy eating and exercise habits developed during saxenda use, as these are key to long-term success.

Mindful eating practices: pay attention to hunger and satiety cues to avoid unconscious overeating.

2. Building a maintenance framework:

Scheduled monitoring: maintain periodic weigh-ins (e.g., weekly or biweekly) to detect early signs of weight regain.

Accountability tools: stay engaged with support systems or digital tools that track behavior and mood.

3. Optional use of lower dose or intermittent therapy:

Bridging strategy: some patients may continue on a lower dose or intermittent use under medical supervision during the early maintenance phase to prevent rebound hunger.

4. Psychological readiness:

Identity shift: embrace your new lifestyle identity—not just someone who lost weight, but someone who lives a healthy, balanced life.

Preventive planning: identify high-risk situations for relapse (e.g., holidays, travel, emotional stress) and develop coping strategies in advance.

SAXENDA FOR SPECIFIC POPULATIONS

Saxenda (liraglutide 3.0 mg), a glp-1 receptor agonist, has become a valuable therapeutic option for chronic weight management in individuals with obesity or overweight with related health conditions. While its efficacy and safety have been established in broad populations, special considerations are necessary when prescribing saxenda to specific groups such as adolescents, women with unique health needs, individuals with coexisting medical conditions, and older adults. This chapter explores the nuanced application of saxenda within these populations, highlighting both clinical insights and practical recommendations.

A. Saxenda use in adolescents: risks and benefits

Fda approval and indications

Saxenda is approved for use in adolescents aged 12 to 17 years with a body weight above 60 kg (132 lbs) and an initial bmi corresponding to ≥30 kg/m² for adults. Its use in this age group reflects increasing concerns about the long-term health implications of adolescent obesity, including early-onset type 2 diabetes, hypertension, and psychosocial challenges.

Clinical benefits

Weight reduction: studies have shown that saxenda can lead to a statistically significant reduction in bmi among adolescents when combined with lifestyle interventions.

Improved metabolic markers: improvements in fasting glucose and insulin sensitivity have been noted, potentially altering the trajectory of metabolic disease in high-risk youth.

Psychological support: weight loss in adolescents may also contribute to improved self-esteem and reduced bullying or social exclusion.

Risks and precautions

Potential for hypoglycemia: while rare, hypoglycemia may occur, particularly in adolescents with coexisting metabolic disorders.

Psychiatric considerations: adolescents are more vulnerable to mood disorders; saxenda's potential to cause suicidal ideation, though rare, requires vigilant monitoring.

Gastrointestinal effects: nausea, vomiting, and reduced appetite are common and may impact adherence in younger patients.

Impact on growth and development: long-term effects on linear growth and pubertal development remain under investigation. Ongoing monitoring is essential.

Clinical guidance:

Use saxenda in adolescents only after comprehensive evaluation, and always in conjunction with behavioral therapy and dietetic support. Close monitoring by pediatric specialists is recommended.

B. Saxenda and women's health (pregnancy, menopause, pcos)

1. Pregnancy and lactation

Contraindicated in pregnancy: saxenda is not recommended during pregnancy due to insufficient data and potential risks. Weight loss offers no benefit during pregnancy and may harm fetal development.

Preconception planning: women of reproductive age should use effective contraception during saxenda treatment and discontinue it at least one month before attempting conception.

Breastfeeding: the safety of saxenda in lactating women is unknown. It is generally advised to avoid use during breastfeeding due to the potential for liraglutide to be excreted in breast milk.

2. Menopause and weight management

Hormonal changes and weight gain: the menopausal transition is often accompanied by an increase in visceral fat and a decline in metabolic rate.

Saxenda's role: liraglutide can help counteract weight gain and metabolic decline in postmenopausal women. It may improve insulin sensitivity and reduce cardiovascular risk factors prevalent in this demographic.

Bone health consideration: some weight loss medications can negatively impact bone density; however, saxenda appears to have a neutral to positive effect, making it a suitable choice in postmenopausal women with osteoporosis risk.

4. Polycystic ovary syndrome (pcos)

Insulin resistance and obesity: pcos is frequently associated with central obesity and insulin resistance. Saxenda has been shown to improve these metabolic parameters in women with pcos.

Menstrual regularity and fertility: preliminary research suggests that weight loss with saxenda may lead to more regular ovulation and improved fertility in women with pcos.

Adjuvant therapy: saxenda can be used alongside metformin and hormonal therapies under medical supervision.

C. Use in patients with coexisting medical conditions

1. Cardiovascular disease (cvd)

Cardioprotective effects: liraglutide has demonstrated cardiovascular benefits in type 2 diabetes populations, reducing the risk of major adverse cardiovascular events (mace). These benefits may extend to saxenda at its higher dose.

Monitoring needs: careful titration and monitoring of heart rate and blood pressure are required, as saxenda can cause an increase in resting heart rate.

Contraindications: patients with unstable angina, recent myocardial infarction, or decompensated heart failure should avoid saxenda.

2. Liver disease

Nafld and nash: saxenda has shown promise in improving hepatic steatosis and inflammatory markers in patients with non-alcoholic fatty liver disease (nafld).

Hepatic impairment: use with caution in patients with moderate hepatic impairment. It is not recommended in those with severe hepatic dysfunction due to a lack of safety data.

3. Kidney disease

Renal considerations: saxenda is not nephrotoxic, but dehydration secondary to gastrointestinal side effects (e.g., vomiting) can precipitate acute kidney injury, particularly in patients with pre-existing renal compromise.

Dose adjustment: no dose adjustment is required in mild to moderate renal impairment, but careful hydration and renal function monitoring are advised.

5. Diabetes mellitus

Type 2 diabetes: while saxenda is distinct from liraglutide 1.8 mg used for glycemic control, its blood sugar-lowering effects can benefit overweight patients with prediabetes or type 2 diabetes.

Medication interactions: avoid concurrent use with other glp-1 receptor agonists or insulin without endocrinology consultation to prevent hypoglycemia.

D. Older adults and saxenda: considerations for safe use

Unique challenges in geriatric populations

Older adults often present with multiple comorbidities, polypharmacy, and age-related physiological changes that affect drug metabolism and sensitivity.

Safety and efficacy

Clinical trials: saxenda has been studied in adults up to age 75. Weight loss benefits are evident, but the response may be slower and side effects more pronounced.

Muscle mass and frailty: weight loss in elderly individuals must be managed carefully to avoid loss of lean muscle mass, which can exacerbate frailty and reduce mobility.

Key considerations:

Start low, go slow: begin with the lowest dose and titrate gradually while monitoring tolerance.

Monitor for dehydration: older adults are more susceptible to dehydration from vomiting or diarrhea, which can lead to falls or acute kidney injury.

Cognitive function: assess for cognitive impairment, as this can impact medication adherence and recognition of side effects.

Functional benefits:

Mobility and independence: modest weight loss can significantly enhance physical function, reduce joint pain, and improve quality of life in older patients.

Cardiometabolic gains: saxenda may aid in reducing cardiovascular risk, improving lipid profiles, and managing blood glucose levels in aging populations.

PSYCHOLOGICAL AND EMOTIONAL ASPECTS OF WEIGHT LOSS

Weight loss is often perceived primarily as a physical journey, focused on diet, exercise, and medication. However, the psychological and emotional dimensions are equally critical—sometimes even more so—especially when using pharmacological aids like saxenda (liraglutide). Understanding and addressing these factors can significantly enhance treatment outcomes, promote lasting change, and improve overall well-being. This chapter explores the complex emotional landscape of weight loss and offers strategies to navigate it effectively.

A. Building a healthy body image

For many individuals embarking on a weight loss journey with saxenda, developing a healthy body image is a profound challenge and an essential goal. Body image refers to how a person perceives, feels about, and relates to their physical appearance. It is shaped by personal beliefs, social messages, and past experiences, and it can be a source of motivation or discouragement.

One common psychological barrier is the internalization of unrealistic or unhealthy beauty ideals. Society often promotes narrow standards of attractiveness, emphasizing thinness or specific body shapes, which can distort self-perception and fuel dissatisfaction. For those with obesity, these ideals can lead to harsh self-criticism, reduced self-esteem, and feelings of inadequacy.

Building a healthy body image means fostering acceptance and respect for the body at every stage of the weight loss process. This includes recognizing the body's strengths and capabilities, appreciating progress beyond the scale, and practicing self-compassion. Mindfulness techniques, such as body scans and affirmations, can help individuals reconnect with their physical selves in a nurturing way. Encouraging patients to set realistic, non-appearance-related goals—such as improved mobility, energy, or emotional resilience—can also shift the focus from aesthetics to holistic health.

Ultimately, cultivating a positive body image supports sustained motivation, reduces emotional eating triggers, and improves mental well-being, thereby complementing the physical effects of saxenda treatment.

B. Overcoming stigma and shame associated with obesity

Weight-related stigma is a pervasive societal issue that profoundly impacts individuals living with obesity. Many face discrimination, judgment, and stereotyping in healthcare settings, workplaces, and social environments. These negative experiences often lead to internalized shame, where people begin to believe and adopt the harsh labels society places on them.

Shame around weight can erode self-worth, exacerbate emotional distress, and lead to maladaptive coping strategies such as binge eating or social withdrawal. It can also discourage individuals from seeking or adhering to treatments like saxenda, fearing judgment or failure.

To overcome stigma and shame, it is crucial to foster an environment of empathy and understanding. Educating patients about the complex biological, psychological, and social factors contributing to obesity helps dismantle simplistic "blame" narratives. Promoting self-compassion practices and affirming the intrinsic value of every individual—regardless of weight—can help counteract shame.

Healthcare providers play a vital role by offering nonjudgmental support, validating patients' struggles, and celebrating their efforts and achievements. Peer support groups can also be powerful spaces for sharing experiences, normalizing challenges, and building collective resilience against stigma.

Addressing stigma and shame not only improves mental health but also enhances engagement with saxenda treatment and promotes healthier, more sustainable lifestyle changes.

C. Using therapy and support groups to enhance results

Weight loss is rarely a purely physical process; emotional and behavioral patterns deeply influence eating habits, activity levels, and self-care. Psychological interventions and social support are critical tools that can enhance the efficacy of saxenda by targeting these underlying factors.

Cognitive behavioral therapy (cbt) is one of the most effective therapeutic approaches in this context. It helps individuals identify and modify distorted thoughts and unhealthy behaviors related to food, body image, and self-esteem. Cbt can also address emotional eating, impulsivity, and stress management, which are common obstacles in weight management.

Other therapeutic modalities, such as acceptance and commitment therapy (act), mindfulness-based therapy, or motivational interviewing, can be integrated depending on individual needs. These therapies encourage emotional acceptance, build intrinsic motivation, and foster adaptive coping mechanisms.

Support groups—whether in-person or online—offer a unique sense of community and accountability. They provide a safe space to share challenges, celebrate milestones, and exchange practical advice. Feeling understood and supported reduces feelings of isolation and shame, which are common in the weight loss journey.

Combining saxenda with therapy and peer support creates a comprehensive approach that addresses both the biological and psychological dimensions of weight management, increasing the likelihood of sustained success.

D. Mental health monitoring during saxenda treatment

Saxenda, like any medication, requires careful monitoring—not only for physical side effects but also for psychological well-being. Some patients may experience changes in mood, anxiety, or emotional regulation during treatment, making mental health monitoring essential.

Clinicians should conduct regular assessments of mood, stress levels, and potential psychiatric symptoms throughout the course of saxenda use. Early identification of issues such as depression or anxiety allows timely intervention and support, preventing treatment discontinuation or complications.

Patients themselves should be encouraged to maintain open communication about their emotional state and to seek professional help if they notice significant mood changes, increased stress, or new psychological symptoms.

A collaborative approach between prescribing physicians, therapists, and patients ensures a balanced treatment plan that promotes both physical weight loss and emotional stability.

E. Creating sustainable motivation and positive habits

Motivation is a dynamic and complex process that fluctuates throughout the weight loss journey. Initial enthusiasm often gives way to challenges, plateaus, or setbacks. Therefore, developing sustainable motivation and cultivating positive habits are critical for long-term success with saxenda.

One key to sustainable motivation is setting clear, realistic, and personally meaningful goals. Rather than focusing solely on weight numbers, goals can include improvements in fitness, energy levels, emotional well-being, or social engagement. Celebrating small wins and progress reinforces positive behavior and builds momentum.

Habit formation is another cornerstone. Replacing unhealthy behaviors with small, manageable actions—such as mindful eating, regular physical activity, or consistent sleep routines—helps embed lifestyle changes into daily life. The use of tools like habit trackers, reminders, or rewards can support this process.

Intrinsic motivation—driven by personal values and internal satisfaction—is more enduring than extrinsic motivation (such as appearance or external praise). Encouraging reflection on why weight loss matters on a deeper level helps patients maintain focus during difficult times.

Combining these psychological strategies with the physiological support of saxenda creates a powerful synergy that not only facilitates weight loss but also builds a foundation for lasting health and well-being.

ALTERNATIVES, SUPPLEMENTS, AND COMPLEMENTARY THERAPIES

In the journey toward effective weight management, saxenda (liraglutide) offers a pharmacological option that has demonstrated significant clinical benefits. However, it is important to recognize that weight loss and maintenance can also be supported or sometimes substituted by various alternative methods, supplements, and complementary therapies. This section explores these options in depth, providing a balanced view to help readers make informed choices alongside or instead of saxenda.

A. Comparing saxenda with natural weight loss supplements

Saxenda is a glucagon-like peptide-1 (glp-1) receptor agonist, prescribed specifically to reduce appetite and enhance satiety by acting on the central nervous system. Its effects are supported by rigorous clinical trials and regulatory approval. In contrast, natural weight loss supplements often rely on herbal extracts, vitamins, minerals, or amino acids purported to influence metabolism, fat absorption, or appetite suppression.

Common natural supplements include green tea extract, garcinia cambogia, conjugated linoleic acid (cla), and fiber supplements. While these may provide mild benefits, their efficacy tends to be inconsistent and generally less potent than saxenda. Furthermore, supplements are not regulated as strictly, leading to variability in quality, dosage, and purity.

It is essential to approach natural supplements with caution. Unlike saxenda, which requires medical supervision, natural supplements can interact unpredictably with medications or health conditions. Therefore, while supplements might serve as adjuncts or initial attempts at weight loss, saxenda's clinical backing and mode of action often make it more suitable for individuals with moderate to severe obesity or those who have struggled with traditional approaches.

    B. Integrating herbal remedies, acupuncture, and lifestyle therapies

Complementary therapies such as herbal remedies and acupuncture have been utilized for centuries across cultures to support weight management, stress reduction, and metabolic health. Herbal remedies like ginger, cinnamon, and fenugreek are believed to aid digestion and reduce inflammation, while acupuncture targets energy meridians purported to influence appetite and hormonal balance.

When integrated thoughtfully with saxenda therapy, these methods may enhance overall wellness and address factors beyond weight alone, such as stress, sleep quality, and emotional eating. Lifestyle therapies remain foundational; dietary modifications, physical activity, and behavioral changes must accompany any pharmacological or complementary approach to yield sustainable results.

Patients considering integrating these therapies should consult with healthcare providers to ensure safety and compatibility with their prescribed treatment plan. Acupuncture, for example, has a low risk profile but requires skilled practitioners to be effective. Herbal remedies should be disclosed to avoid potential interactions. Ultimately, the synergy of medical treatment and holistic care can offer a more comprehensive path to weight management.

C. When to consider bariatric surgery instead

Bariatric surgery remains the most effective intervention for significant and sustained weight loss in individuals with severe obesity or obesity-related comorbidities. Surgery options, such as gastric bypass, sleeve gastrectomy, or adjustable gastric banding, produce physiological changes that restrict food intake and/or alter nutrient absorption.

While saxenda can help many patients reduce weight and improve metabolic health, it may be insufficient for those with a body mass index (bmi) over 40 or those with bmi over 35 who have serious conditions like type 2 diabetes, hypertension, or sleep apnea.

Referral for bariatric surgery evaluation is appropriate when conservative management—including lifestyle, pharmacotherapy (such as saxenda), and behavioral therapies—fails to produce adequate weight loss or improve health markers. Surgery carries higher upfront risks and requires lifelong nutritional monitoring, but it often yields dramatic improvements in weight and comorbidities.

Patients should engage in a thorough discussion with bariatric specialists to weigh benefits, risks, and lifestyle changes before opting for surgery. For many, saxenda represents an important step in a graduated approach to obesity treatment, with surgery reserved for more severe or refractory cases.

D.   Combining saxenda with cognitive behavioral therapy

Cognitive behavioral therapy (cbt) is a well-established psychological intervention that addresses patterns of thought and behavior contributing to unhealthy eating, sedentary lifestyle, and weight gain. When combined with saxenda, cbt can significantly enhance treatment outcomes by helping patients develop coping strategies, improve motivation, and maintain behavioral changes critical for long-term success.

Cbt focuses on identifying and restructuring cognitive distortions, emotional triggers, and environmental factors that lead to overeating or inactivity. Through structured sessions with trained therapists, patients learn to set realistic goals, manage cravings, and build a positive relationship with food and body image.

Clinical studies have shown that pharmacotherapy combined with cbt is more effective in producing sustained weight loss than either approach alone. Saxenda helps reduce physiological hunger signals, while cbt empowers patients psychologically to maintain healthier habits beyond the pharmacological effects.

Incorporating cbt into a comprehensive weight management program alongside saxenda is highly recommended, especially for individuals with emotional or binge eating tendencies, or those who have experienced repeated dieting failures.

E. Evaluating long-term options for weight management

Weight management is a lifelong endeavor. While saxenda can be effective for initial weight loss and maintenance, patients and healthcare providers must plan for sustainable strategies that adapt over time. This includes monitoring for diminishing pharmacological effects, managing side effects, and adjusting treatment as needed.

Long-term options may involve continued use of saxenda under medical supervision, transitioning to other pharmacotherapies if indicated, or shifting emphasis toward intensive lifestyle modification supported by behavioral therapy. Additionally, ongoing assessment of metabolic health, psychological well-being, and quality of life is critical.

Patients should also be aware of the potential need to cycle treatments or combine therapies for optimal results. Alternative and complementary approaches discussed earlier may play a role in maintaining weight loss and preventing regain.

Ultimately, the choice of long-term strategy should be personalized, flexible, and patient-centered, emphasizing realistic goals, self-efficacy, and support systems. Regular follow-up with healthcare professionals ensures that adjustments can be made proactively, maximizing the chance of durable success.

REAL STORIES AND EXPERT PERSPECTIVES

The journey with saxenda, like any weight management treatment, is as much about individual experience as it is about clinical guidance. This section delves into the authentic voices of patients, the expertise of medical professionals, and the collective wisdom of the saxenda community. By weaving together personal testimonials, expert insights, frequently asked questions, and detailed case studies, we aim to offer a holistic view of what it means to use saxenda effectively and responsibly. Whether you're just beginning or have been on the medication for a while, these stories and perspectives provide support, knowledge, and inspiration.

A. Patient testimonials: successes and challenges

The heart of any treatment lies in the real-life experiences of those who have taken it. Patient testimonials illuminate the highs and lows of saxenda use, reminding us that weight management is a complex, personal, and ongoing journey.

Successes:

Many users report significant positive changes in both their physical and emotional health. Jessica, a 42-year-old mother of two, shares:

"after years of struggling with weight, saxenda helped me shed 15 kilograms in six months. More than the numbers, i regained my energy and confidence. Everyday activities no longer exhaust me. The support from my healthcare provider combined with saxenda made a real difference."

Similarly, michael, a 55-year-old office worker, highlights how saxenda helped break his cycle of emotional eating:

"the medication reduced my appetite, but it also gave me space to rebuild healthier habits. I didn't just lose weight— i changed how i relate to food."

Challenges:

While success stories are inspiring, it is important to recognize the challenges faced by many users. Common side effects such as nausea, headaches, or mild gastrointestinal discomfort can test patience and perseverance. Sarah explains:

"the first few weeks were tough. Nausea hit me hard, and i worried i wouldn't be able to continue. But with gradual dose adjustments and guidance from my doctor, i learned to manage it."

Others note that weight loss plateaus and emotional struggles can sometimes dampen motivation. These testimonials highlight the need for patience, realistic expectations, and comprehensive support beyond medication alone.

B. Insights from endocrinologists and obesity specialists

Endocrinologists and obesity specialists offer invaluable clinical context to saxenda's role in weight management. Their perspectives emphasize that saxenda is one tool within a broader treatment plan tailored to each individual's unique physiology and lifestyle.

Dr. Anita kumar, an endocrinologist with over 15 years of experience, explains:

"saxenda is a glucagon-like peptide-1 (glp-1) receptor agonist that helps regulate appetite and energy balance. It's important to understand that this medication works best when combined with lifestyle changes like diet and exercise. Patients often see the most sustained results when saxenda is part of a multidisciplinary approach."

Obesity specialist dr. Miguel hernandez highlights patient selection and monitoring:

"not everyone is a candidate for saxenda. We evaluate medical history, weight-related health risks, and psychological readiness. Close follow-up is critical to manage side effects and adjust dosages. Long-term adherence and support are keys to success."

Both experts emphasize that saxenda is not a quick fix but a component of a sustained commitment to health. They also underline the importance of mental health support, given the emotional challenges many patients face during their weight loss journey.

C. Frequently asked questions from the saxenda community

Across forums, support groups, and clinical visits, certain questions consistently arise. These faqs provide clarity and reassurance based on the collective experiences of the saxenda community:

1. How soon can i expect to see results?

Many users notice appetite suppression within the first few weeks, but meaningful weight loss typically appears after 4–6 weeks. Patience is crucial.

2. What are the most common side effects, and how can i manage them?

Nausea, vomiting, diarrhea, and constipation are common initially. Gradual dose escalation and hydration can help. If symptoms persist, consult your healthcare provider.

3. Can i stop taking saxenda once i reach my goal weight?

Stopping saxenda may lead to weight regain if lifestyle changes are not firmly established. Long-term maintenance often requires ongoing treatment and behavioral modifications.

4. Is saxenda safe with other medications?

Discuss all medications and supplements with your doctor to avoid interactions, especially for diabetes, blood pressure, or thyroid medications.

5. How does saxenda affect mental health?

Some users report mood changes. It is important to monitor emotional well-being and seek support if anxiety or depression symptoms arise.

D. Case studies on weight loss journeys with saxenda

Case studies offer a detailed look into the multifaceted nature of weight management with saxenda. These narratives provide lessons on what can work, what to expect, and how individualized each journey can be.

Case study 1: anna's gradual transformation

Anna, age 38, struggled with obesity-related fatigue and prediabetes. Under medical supervision, she began saxenda with a slow dose escalation. Over 12 months, she lost 25 kg and improved her blood sugar levels significantly. Key factors included her commitment to a mediterranean diet and daily walks. Challenges included managing mild nausea early on and overcoming a mid-treatment weight plateau through behavioral therapy.

Case study 2: david's emotional eating challenge

David, a 45-year-old, battled emotional eating triggered by work stress. Saxenda helped reduce his hunger cues, but relapse occurred during stressful periods. With the addition of cognitive-behavioral therapy and mindfulness practices, david regained control and lost 18 kg in 10 months. His case underscores the importance of addressing psychological factors alongside pharmacotherapy.

Case study 3: maria's experience with side effects

Maria, 52, experienced significant gastrointestinal side effects initially, leading to temporary discontinuation. After restarting with a slower dose increase and dietary adjustments, she found better tolerance and eventually lost 12 kg. Her persistence demonstrates the value of personalized dosing schedules and close provider communication.

E. Encouragement from long-term users

Long-term users of saxenda provide hope and encouragement to newcomers, emphasizing perseverance, self-compassion, and holistic health.

Jessica, who has been on saxenda for over two years, advises:

"this is not just a medication; it's a journey of learning your body and being patient with yourself. Celebrate every small victory and remember that setbacks don't define you."

Carlos, another long-term user, reflects on lifestyle change:

"saxenda gave me the initial push, but the real change came when i embraced exercise and mindful eating. It's about balance, not perfection."

Their voices remind us that sustainable weight management is a marathon, not a sprint. Consistency, support, and realistic goals are the foundation for lasting success.

CONCLUSION

A. Recap of saxenda's role in weight management

Throughout this guide, we have explored saxenda as a scientifically supported tool designed to assist individuals on their weight management journey. Saxenda's active ingredient, liraglutide, works by mimicking a natural hormone that helps regulate appetite, reduce food intake, and ultimately support gradual, sustainable weight loss. While not a magic pill or a standalone solution, saxenda is an important component of a comprehensive approach that includes healthy nutrition, regular physical activity, and behavioral changes. Understanding its role—and limitations—is key to setting realistic expectations and achieving meaningful, lasting results.

B. Empowering informed and safe usage

A cornerstone of successful saxenda therapy is knowledge and vigilance. This guide has emphasized the importance of informed usage: starting at the correct dosage, adhering to prescribed instructions, monitoring side effects, and maintaining regular communication with healthcare providers. Empowerment comes from being proactive—recognizing how your body responds, asking questions, and addressing concerns early. Saxenda's effectiveness depends not just on the medication itself but on the partnership between patient and provider. Safety is paramount, and by following best practices, users can maximize benefits while minimizing risks.

C. Long-term vision for health beyond the medication

Saxenda is a valuable aid, but it is not an endpoint. The ultimate goal transcends the numbers on the scale; it is about embracing a healthier lifestyle that supports physical, mental, and emotional well-being for the long term. This means cultivating sustainable habits—balanced eating, consistent activity, stress management, and self-care—that persist even after medication is discontinued. Viewing saxenda as a catalyst rather than a cure empowers users to take ownership of their health journey. The transformation begins with weight loss, but the true success lies in holistic, lifelong wellness.

D.   Final words: you're more than a number on the scale

It is essential to remember that your worth, identity, and happiness are not defined solely by your weight or appearance. Weight management is deeply personal and often complex, involving biological, psychological, and social factors. This guide recognizes that struggle and encourages compassion toward oneself throughout the process. Celebrate progress in all its forms—improved energy, better sleep, increased confidence, or enhanced mobility—not just pounds lost. You are a whole person with a unique story, and saxenda is simply one chapter in your journey toward a healthier, more fulfilling life.

E. Resources, support networks, and next steps

As you close this book, know that support is available every step of the way. Whether through healthcare professionals, registered dietitians, counseling services, or peer support groups, connecting with others can provide motivation, accountability, and shared understanding. Additionally, various online communities and educational platforms offer ongoing resources to deepen your knowledge and inspire your commitment. Your next steps might include scheduling regular follow-ups, refining your meal and exercise plans, or seeking mental health support if needed. Remember, sustained success is rarely a solitary pursuit—embrace the network around you and keep moving forward with confidence.

THE END

www.ingramcontent.com/pod-product-compliance
Ingram Content Group UK Ltd.
Pitfield, Milton Keynes, MK11 3LW, UK
UKHW060756201025
8476UKWH00027B/502